WHAT SHORTENS LIVES?

Understanding Life-Shortening Factors and Effective Remedies for All

SAMUEL EKPENYONG

WHAT SHORTENS LIVES?

Published by: Samek Books ®

ISBN: 9798335612807

samuelekpenyong.mkd@gmail.com

www.amazon.com/author/samek-books

Cover Designer: Shae Coon, Texas.

bookdesignsbyshae@gmail.com

FOREWORD

In the quest to understand and combat the myriad factors that contribute to reduced lifespan, Samuel Ekpenyong's work, "What Shortens Lives? Understanding Life-Shortening Factors and Effective Remedies for All," stands out as a pivotal contribution. This comprehensive exploration of life-shortening factors is not only timely but essential, providing both depth and clarity on a subject that affects every individual.

Samuel Ekpenyong's rigorous analysis and insightful approach illuminate the complex interplay between genetic, environmental, and lifestyle factors that contribute to diminished longevity. His ability to distill complex scientific concepts into actionable knowledge underscores the significance of this work. It reflects a profound understanding of the challenges we face and offers practical, evidence-based remedies to address them.

As a scholar and practitioner in public health, I appreciate the meticulous attention to detail and the balanced perspective presented in this volume. Ekpenyong's contributions are especially valuable in an era where informed decisions and preventive measures are crucial to enhancing life quality and extending lifespan. This book is not only a significant academic achievement but also a practical guide that can inform both policy and personal health choices.

I wholeheartedly recommend this book to researchers, healthcare professionals, and anyone interested in the factors influencing longevity. Samuel Ekpenyong's work is a testament to his dedication and expertise in the field, and it promises to be an influential resource in advancing our understanding and application of life-extending strategies.

Dr. Emily Jones

Professor of Epidemiology

University of Oxford

TABLE OF CONTENTS

PREFACE

In today's rapidly evolving world of health and wellness, understanding the multifaceted factors that impact longevity is more important than ever. "What Shortens Lives?" is designed to be your comprehensive guide to navigating the complex landscape of health risks and remedies.

As our knowledge of health continues to advance, it becomes increasingly crucial to grasp how various factors—ranging from chronic diseases and lifestyle choices to environmental influences and genetic predispositions—affect our overall well-being. This book aims to bridge the gap between complex scientific research and practical, actionable advice, providing readers with a thorough understanding of how to improve and extend their lives.

In crafting this book, my goal was to offer a resource that is not only informative but also empowering. Each chapter delves into critical aspects of health and longevity, presenting evidence-based insights and practical strategies that can be applied universally. From managing chronic diseases and overcoming substance use to addressing environmental hazards and optimizing mental health, this book covers a wide range of topics relevant to everyone.

By exploring these life-shortening factors and effective remedies, "What Shortens Lives?" equips readers with the knowledge needed to make informed decisions about their health. Whether you are an individual seeking to enhance your well-being or a healthcare professional aiming to provide better care, this book offers valuable guidance for achieving a healthier, more fulfilling life.

I invite you to engage with the content and explore the strategies provided. By integrating the insights and recommendations from this book into your daily life, you can take proactive steps towards a longer, healthier future.

Warm regards,

Samuel Ekpenyong

CHAPTER ONE

INTRODUCTION: UNDERSTANDING LIFE-SHORTENING FACTORS

Life expectancy, the average period a person is expected to live, is influenced by a multitude of factors, encompassing both modifiable and non-modifiable elements. Several key factors have been identified as contributing to a reduction in lifespan. These include lifestyle choices, chronic diseases, mental health conditions, substance use, environmental exposures, and genetic predispositions.

DEFINITIONS AND KEY CONCEPTS

Life Expectancy

Life expectancy is a statistical measure indicating the average number of years a person is expected to live based on current mortality rates. It is a critical indicator of a population's overall health and well-being. Factors influencing life expectancy include access to healthcare, socioeconomic conditions, and lifestyle choices.

Morbidity vs. Mortality

• Morbidity refers to the presence of illness or disease. Chronic morbid conditions such as diabetes and hypertension can negatively impact quality of life and potentially shorten lifespan.

• Mortality is the state of being subject to death. Mortality rates are used to measure the frequency of deaths in a population, often segmented by age, gender, and cause.

Risk Factors

Risk factors are characteristics or behaviors that increase the likelihood of developing a disease or health condition. These can be categorized into:

- Modifiable Risk Factors: Lifestyle choices such as diet, physical activity, smoking, and alcohol consumption.

- Non-Modifiable Risk Factors: Genetic predispositions, age, and sex.

Comorbidity

Comorbidity refers to the occurrence of two or more diseases or conditions simultaneously in an individual. The presence of multiple comorbid conditions often exacerbates health issues and can lead to a compounded reduction in life expectancy.

MAJOR CATEGORIES OF LIFE-SHORTENING FACTORS

Lifestyle Choices

- Diet: Poor dietary habits, including high intake of processed foods, saturated fats, and sugars, are associated with increased risk of chronic diseases such as cardiovascular disease, diabetes, and obesity.

- Physical Activity: Sedentary lifestyles are linked to a higher risk of obesity, cardiovascular diseases, and certain cancers. Regular physical activity is crucial for maintaining cardiovascular health, muscle strength, and overall longevity.

Chronic Diseases

- Cardiovascular Disease: Includes conditions such as heart disease and hypertension, which are significant contributors to premature mortality. These conditions are often influenced by lifestyle factors such as diet and physical activity.

- Diabetes: A chronic metabolic disorder characterized by high blood sugar levels. Diabetes increases the risk of heart disease, stroke, and kidney failure, all of which can shorten lifespan.

Mental Health

- Stress: Chronic stress has been shown to contribute to a range of health issues, including cardiovascular disease and weakened immune function.

- Depression: Clinical depression affects both mental and physical health, leading to poor health outcomes and an increased risk of mortality.

Substance Use

- Smoking: Tobacco use is a major risk factor for numerous health problems, including lung cancer, cardiovascular disease, and respiratory disorders. Smoking significantly reduces life expectancy.

- Alcohol and Drug Abuse: Excessive alcohol consumption and illicit drug use can lead to liver disease, cardiovascular problems, and increased risk of accidents and violence.

Environmental Factors

- Pollution: Exposure to environmental pollutants such as air and water pollution has been linked to respiratory and cardiovascular diseases, which can adversely affect longevity.

- Hazardous Living Conditions: Poor living conditions, including inadequate sanitation and exposure to harmful chemicals, can negatively impact health.

Genetic Factors

- Genetic Predisposition: Certain genetic traits can increase susceptibility to diseases such as cancer and heart disease. While genetic factors are not modifiable, their impact can be mitigated through lifestyle changes and medical interventions.

IMPORTANCE OF ADDRESSING LIFE-SHORTENING FACTORS

Addressing and mitigating life-shortening factors is essential for enhancing quality of life and extending lifespan. By understanding and managing these factors, individuals can make informed decisions that promote long-term health and well-being. Through preventive measures, such as healthy lifestyle choices and regular medical check-ups, it is possible to significantly reduce the risk of premature mortality and improve overall health outcomes.

In the subsequent chapters, we will explore these factors in greater detail, providing evidence-based insights and practical strategies to counteract their effects and promote a healthier, longer life.

CHAPTER TWO

LIFESTYLE CHOICES: THE IMPACT OF DIET AND EXERCISE

THE ROLE OF DIET IN LONGEVITY

Nutritional Fundamentals

Dietary habits play a pivotal role in determining overall health and longevity. Nutrition involves the intake and utilization of essential nutrients required for maintaining bodily functions and overall health. Key nutrients include:

- Macronutrients: Carbohydrates, proteins, and fats are required in large amounts and provide energy, support growth, and repair tissues.

- Micronutrients: Vitamins and minerals are

needed in smaller amounts but are crucial for various biochemical processes and preventing deficiencies.

Impact of Poor Dietary Habits

- Obesity: Excessive caloric intake, particularly from high-fat and high-sugar foods, contributes to obesity. Obesity is associated with a higher risk of developing chronic diseases such as type 2 diabetes, cardiovascular disease, and certain cancers. According to the World Health Organization (WHO), obesity significantly reduces life expectancy and quality of life.

- Cardiovascular Health: Diets high in saturated fats, trans fats, and cholesterol can lead to the buildup of plaques in arteries, increasing the risk of heart disease and stroke. The American Heart Association recommends a diet rich in fruits, vegetables, whole grains, and lean proteins to mitigate these risks.

- Diabetes: High intake of refined carbohydrates and sugary foods can lead to insulin resistance and type 2 diabetes. Proper management of carbohydrate intake, along with a balanced diet, is essential for controlling blood sugar levels.

Evidence-Based Dietary Recommendations

- Mediterranean Diet: Rich in fruits, vegetables, whole grains, nuts, and olive oil, and low in red meat, this diet has been associated with reduced risk of cardiovascular disease and longer lifespan.

- DASH Diet (Dietary Approaches to Stop Hypertension): Emphasizes fruits, vegetables, whole grains, and lean proteins while reducing salt intake. It is effective in lowering blood pressure and promoting heart health.

The Role of Physical Activity in Longevity

Benefits of Regular Exercise

Physical activity is a critical component of a healthy lifestyle. Regular exercise offers numerous benefits, including:

> Cardiovascular Health: Engaging in aerobic activities such as walking, running, or cycling improves cardiovascular health by strengthening the heart and improving circulation.

> Weight Management: Exercise helps regulate body weight by balancing energy expenditure and caloric intake. It also promotes muscle mass, which aids in metabolism.

> Mental Health: Physical activity has been shown to reduce symptoms of depression and anxiety. It stimulates

the release of endorphins, which are known as "feel-good" hormones.

Longevity: Studies consistently show that regular physical activity is associated with a lower risk of premature mortality. For instance, the American College of Sports Medicine recommends at least 150 minutes of moderate-intensity aerobic exercise per week to maintain health and prevent chronic diseases.

Types of Exercise and Their Benefits

• Aerobic Exercise: Activities like running, swimming, and cycling improve cardiovascular fitness and endurance.

• Strength Training: Exercises such as weight lifting and resistance training build muscle mass, support bone health, and enhance metabolic function.

• Flexibility and Balance: Activities like yoga and stretching improve flexibility, balance, and overall mobility, reducing the risk of falls and injuries.

Guidelines for Incorporating Exercise

1. Frequency: Aim for at least 150 minutes of moderate-intensity aerobic activity per week, combined with muscle-strengthening activities on two or more days per week.

2. Intensity: Exercise intensity should be adjusted based on individual fitness levels. A combination of moderate and vigorous activities is recommended for optimal health benefits.

3. Consistency: Consistency is key to reaping the long-term benefits of exercise. Establishing a regular exercise routine and gradually increasing intensity and duration can lead to sustained health improvements.

Integrating Healthy Diet and Exercise Habits

Creating a Balanced Lifestyle Plan

To maximize health benefits and extend lifespan, it is crucial to integrate healthy eating and regular exercise into daily life. This can be achieved by:

Setting Realistic Goals: Establish achievable dietary and exercise goals that can be gradually integrated into daily routines.

Monitoring Progress: Keep track of dietary intake and physical activity to ensure adherence to health goals and make adjustments as needed.

Seeking Professional Guidance: Consulting with healthcare providers, such as dietitians and fitness trainers, can help tailor a personalized plan that addresse Seeking Professional

Guidance: Consulting with healthcare providers, such as dietitians and fitness trainers, can help tailor a personalized plan that addresses individual needs and health conditions.

Overcoming Barriers

Addressing common barriers to maintaining a healthy lifestyle, such as time constraints, lack of motivation, and limited access to resources, can enhance adherence to diet and exercise plans. Practical solutions include meal planning, incorporating physical activity into daily routines, and seeking support from community resources.

In summary, diet and exercise are fundamental components of a healthy lifestyle and play a significant role in determining longevity. Adopting a balanced diet rich in essential nutrients and engaging in regular physical activity can substantially reduce the risk of chronic diseases, improve overall health, and extend life expectancy. By understanding and implementing evidence-based dietary and exercise recommendations, individuals can make informed choices that promote a longer, healthier life.

CHAPTER THREE

CHRONIC DISEASES: MANAGING AND PREVENTING MAJOR HEALTH CONDITIONS

UNDERSTANDING CHRONIC DISEASES

Definition and Characteristics

Chronic diseases are long-lasting conditions that often develop slowly over time and persist for months or years. They are typically characterized by:

- Prolonged Duration: Chronic diseases generally last for a long time, often for the remainder of an individual's life.

- Slow Onset: Symptoms may develop gradually and may not be

immediately apparent.

- Impact on Daily Life: These conditions can affect daily activities and quality of life, requiring ongoing management and treatment.

Prevalence and Impact

Chronic diseases are leading causes of morbidity and mortality worldwide. According to the World Health Organization (WHO), chronic diseases account for approximately 71% of global deaths. They include conditions such as cardiovascular disease, diabetes, chronic respiratory diseases, and cancer.

CARDIOVASCULAR DISEASE

Cardiovascular disease (CVD) encompasses a range of conditions affecting the heart and blood vessels, including coronary artery disease, heart failure, and stroke. It is a leading cause of death globally.

Risk Factors

Hypertension: High blood pressure can damage arterial walls, leading to atherosclerosis (buildup of plaques in arteries) and increasing the risk of heart attack and stroke.

Hyperlipidemia: Elevated levels of cholesterol and triglycerides in the blood contribute to plaque formation and cardiovascular disease.

Lifestyle Factors: Poor diet, lack of physical activity, smoking, and excessive alcohol consumption are significant risk factors for CVD.

Management and Prevention

- Lifestyle Modifications: Adopting a heart-healthy diet, engaging in regular physical activity, quitting smoking, and reducing alcohol intake are crucial for managing and preventing CVD.

- Medical Interventions: Medications such as statins and antihypertensives, and in some cases, surgical interventions like angioplasty or bypass surgery, may be necessary.

Diabetes Mellitus

Diabetes mellitus is a metabolic disorder characterized by chronic hyperglycemia (high blood sugar levels). The two main types are type 1 diabetes (an autoimmune condition) and type 2 diabetes (often associated with lifestyle factors).

Risk Factors

Obesity: Excess body fat, particularly abdominal fat, is a major risk factor for type 2 diabetes.

Genetics: Family history and genetic predispositions can increase the risk of developing diabetes.

Sedentary Lifestyle: Lack of physical activity contributes to insulin resistance and the development of diabetes.

Management and Prevention

- Diet and Exercise: A balanced diet, low in refined carbohydrates and high in fiber, combined with regular physical activity, is essential for managing and preventing diabetes.

- Medication: Oral hypoglycemic agents or insulin therapy may be required to control blood sugar levels.

- Monitoring: Regular monitoring of blood glucose levels and maintaining a healthy weight are important for diabetes management.

CHRONIC RESPIRATORY DISEASES

Chronic respiratory diseases, including chronic obstructive pulmonary disease (COPD) and asthma, affect the airways and lung tissue, leading to breathing difficulties.

Risk Factors

Smoking: The primary cause of COPD, smoking damages the airways and lung tissue, leading to reduced lung function.

Environmental Exposures: Long-term exposure to air pollutants and occupational hazards can contribute to chronic respiratory diseases.

Management and Prevention

- Smoking Cessation: Quitting smoking is the most effective way to prevent and manage COPD and improve respiratory health.

- Medication: Inhalers and other medications can help manage symptoms and improve lung function.

- Avoiding Triggers: Reducing exposure to allergens and irritants can help manage asthma and other respiratory conditions.

CANCER

Cancer encompasses a diverse group of diseases characterized by uncontrolled cell growth and spread to other parts of the body. Common types include lung cancer, prostate cancer, and colorectal cancer.

Risk Factors

Lifestyle Factors: Smoking, excessive alcohol consumption, and poor diet are significant risk factors for various types of cancer.

Genetic Factors: Certain genetic mutations can increase the risk of developing cancer. For example, BRCA1 and BRCA2 gene mutations are associated with higher risks of breast and ovarian cancers.

Management and Prevention

Screening: Regular screening and early detection are crucial for effective treatment and improved outcomes.

Lifestyle Modifications: A healthy diet,

regular exercise, and avoiding known carcinogens are essential for reducing cancer risk.

Medical Interventions: Treatment options vary based on cancer type and stage and may include surgery, radiation therapy, chemotherapy, and targeted therapies.

COMPREHENSIVE STRATEGIES FOR CHRONIC DISEASE MANAGEMENT

Integrated Approach

An integrated approach to managing chronic diseases involves a combination of lifestyle changes, medical treatment, and regular monitoring. Key components include:

- Multidisciplinary Care: Collaboration among healthcare providers, including primary care physicians, specialists, dietitians, and mental health professionals, ensures comprehensive management of chronic conditions.

- Patient Education: Educating patients about their conditions, treatment options, and lifestyle modifications is essential for effective self-management and adherence to treatment plans.

HEALTH PROMOTION AND PREVENTIVE MEASURES

Promoting overall health and preventing chronic diseases requires proactive measures, including:

Health Education: Public health campaigns and educational programs can raise awareness about chronic disease prevention and management.

Policy and Environmental Changes: Implementing policies that promote healthy environments, such as reducing tobacco use and improving access to healthy foods, can help prevent chronic diseases at the population level.

Conclusion

Chronic diseases significantly impact health and longevity, but their effects can be mitigated through effective management and prevention strategies. By understanding the risk factors and adopting evidence-based approaches to treatment and lifestyle modification, individuals can improve their quality of life and extend their lifespan. The next chapters will explore the role of mental health, substance use, environmental factors, and genetics in health outcomes and provide strategies for addressing these issues to promote a longer, healthier life.

CHAPTER FOUR

MENTAL HEALTH: THE HIDDEN IMPACT OF STRESS AND DEPRESSION

DEFINITION AND SCOPE

Mental health encompasses emotional, psychological, and social well-being. It affects how individuals think, feel, and act, and plays a crucial role in determining how they handle stress, relate to others, and make decisions. Good mental health is integral to overall well-being and longevity. Mental health issues, including stress and depression, can have profound impacts on physical health and life expectancy.

The biopsychosocial model of mental health emphasizes the interplay between biological, psychological, and social factors. This model recognizes that mental health is influenced by genetics, brain chemistry, personal experiences, and social environment. Effective management of mental health involves addressing these interconnected aspects.

THE IMPACT OF STRESS ON HEALTH

Understanding Stress

Stress is a physiological and psychological response to perceived threats or demands. It can be acute (short-term) or chronic (long-term). While acute stress can be motivating, chronic stress can have detrimental effects on health.

Physiological Effects

- Cardiovascular System: Chronic stress can lead to elevated blood pressure and increased risk of heart disease. The release of stress hormones like cortisol and adrenaline can contribute to hypertension and arterial damage.

- Immune System: Prolonged stress can suppress immune function, making individuals more susceptible to infections and illnesses.

- Metabolism: Stress can lead to changes in metabolism, contributing to weight gain, obesity, and insulin resistance.

Psychological and Behavioral Effects

- Mental Health Disorders: Chronic stress is associated with higher risks of anxiety disorders, depression, and other mental health issues.

- Behavioral Changes: Stress can lead to unhealthy behaviors such as poor diet, substance abuse, and lack of physical activity, further exacerbating health problems.

Management Strategies

- Stress Reduction Techniques: Techniques such as mindfulness meditation, deep breathing exercises, and progressive muscle relaxation can help manage stress.

- Lifestyle Adjustments: Regular physical activity, adequate sleep, and a balanced diet are essential for stress management.

- Professional Support: Cognitive-behavioral therapy (CBT) and other therapeutic approaches can be effective in addressing chronic stress.

DEPRESSION: CAUSES, SYMPTOMS, AND EFFECTS

Understanding Depression

Depression, or major depressive disorder (MDD), is a mental health condition characterized by persistent feelings of sadness, hopelessness, and loss of interest in activities. It affects daily functioning and quality of life.

CAUSES AND RISK FACTORS

1. Biological Factors: Neurochemical imbalances, genetic predispositions, and hormonal changes can contribute to the development of depression.

2. Psychological Factors: Cognitive patterns, such as negative thinking and low self-esteem, play a role in depression.

3. Social Factors: Stressful life events, social isolation, and lack of support networks can

increase the risk of depression.

SYMPTOMS

Common symptoms of depression include:

Persistent feelings of sadness or emptiness

Loss of interest in previously enjoyed activities

Changes in appetite or weight

Sleep disturbances

Fatigue and loss of energy

Difficulty concentrating

Thoughts of death or suicide

EFFECTS ON PHYSICAL HEALTH

1. Cardiovascular Health: Depression is associated with an increased risk of cardiovascular disease and stroke.

2. Immune System: Depression can weaken the immune system, making individuals more susceptible to illness.

3. Chronic Conditions: Depression can exacerbate chronic conditions like diabetes and arthritis, leading to poorer health outcomes.

Management and Treatment

• **Medication:** Antidepressants, such as selective serotonin reuptake inhibitors (SSRIs) and serotonin-norepinephrine reuptake inhibitors (SNRIs), can be effective in managing depression.

• **Psychotherapy**: Cognitive-behavioral therapy (CBT) and other forms of psychotherapy can help individuals address negative thought patterns and develop coping strategies.

• **Lifestyle Changes**: Regular physical

activity, healthy eating, and establishing a routine can improve mood and overall well-being.

THE ROLE OF SOCIAL SUPPORT

Importance of Social Connections

Social support plays a critical role in mental health. Strong social connections can provide emotional support, reduce feelings of isolation, and enhance resilience against stress.

Building Support Networks

• Family and Friends: Maintaining relationships with family and friends can offer emotional comfort and practical assistance.

• Community Engagement: Participating in community activities and support groups can foster a sense of belonging and reduce isolation.

• Professional Help: Engaging with mental health professionals can provide additional support and resources for managing mental health issues.

PREVENTIVE MEASURES AND HEALTH PROMOTION

Early Intervention

Early identification and intervention for mental health issues can prevent the progression of conditions like stress and depression. Regular mental health check-ups and seeking help at the first signs of trouble are crucial for effective management.

Promoting Mental Well-Being

Education and Awareness: Raising awareness about mental health and reducing stigma can encourage individuals to seek help and adopt preventive measures.

Healthy Lifestyle: Integrating practices such as stress management techniques, healthy eating, and regular exercise into daily life can promote mental well-being.

Conclusion

Mental health significantly impacts overall health and longevity. Chronic stress and depression can have profound effects on physical health, contributing to a range of chronic conditions and reducing life expectancy. By understanding the effects of mental health issues and implementing effective management strategies, individuals can improve their quality of life and promote a longer, healthier life. The subsequent chapters will explore additional factors affecting health, including substance use, environmental influences, and genetic predispositions, providing a comprehensive approach to health and longevity.

CHAPTER FIVE

SUBSTANCE USE: THE RISKS OF SMOKING, ALCOHOL, AND DRUG USE

INTRODUCTION TO SUBSTANCE USE

Substance use, encompassing smoking, alcohol consumption, and drug use, is a significant factor influencing health and longevity. These substances can have both short-term and long-term effects on physical and mental health, contributing to various health conditions and reducing life expectancy.

Definitions and Key Concepts

Substance Use Disorder (SUD): A

medical condition characterized by an inability to control the use of substances, leading to significant impairment or distress. It includes dependence and addiction.

Addiction: A chronic, relapsing disorder characterized by compulsive drug-seeking behavior and continued use despite harmful consequences.

THE RISKS OF SMOKING

Smoking is the leading cause of preventable death worldwide. It involves the inhalation of tobacco smoke, which contains numerous harmful chemicals, including nicotine, tar, and carbon monoxide.

Health Impacts

- Respiratory System: Smoking damages the respiratory tract, leading to chronic bronchitis, emphysema, and chronic obstructive pulmonary disease (COPD). It also significantly increases the risk of lung cancer.

- Cardiovascular System: Tobacco use contributes to the development of atherosclerosis (plaque buildup in arteries), which can lead to coronary artery disease, stroke, and hypertension.

- Overall Health: Smoking weakens the immune system, increases susceptibility to infections, and accelerates the aging process, contributing to premature mortality.

Quitting Smoking

- Health Benefits: Quitting smoking leads to immediate and long-term health benefits, including reduced risks of cardiovascular disease, improved lung function, and lower cancer risk.

- Strategies: Effective smoking cessation strategies include nicotine replacement therapies (patches, gums), prescription medications (varenicline, bupropion), and behavioral therapies.

THE RISKS OF ALCOHOL USE

Alcohol use can range from moderate consumption to excessive and problematic use. While moderate alcohol consumption may have some perceived health benefits, excessive use leads to numerous health risks.

Health Impacts

- Liver Disease: Chronic alcohol consumption can lead to liver conditions such as fatty liver disease, hepatitis, and cirrhosis.

- Cardiovascular Health: Excessive alcohol

use increases the risk of hypertension, cardiomyopathy, and arrhythmias. It also contributes to stroke and heart disease.

- Mental Health: Heavy alcohol use can exacerbate mental health issues such as depression and anxiety, and impair cognitive function and judgment.

- Cancer: Alcohol consumption is a known risk factor for several types of cancer, including mouth, throat, esophagus, liver, colon, and breast cancer.

Moderation and Treatment

- Moderation: The recommended guidelines suggest no more than one drink per day for women and two drinks per day for men.

- Treatment: For individuals with alcohol use disorder, treatment options include counseling, behavioral therapies, and medications such as disulfiram, naltrexone, and acamprosate.

THE RISKS OF DRUG USE

Drug use includes both the misuse of prescription medications and the use of illicit drugs. Both types of drug use can lead to severe health consequences.

Health Impacts

- Physical Health: Illicit drugs such as heroin, cocaine, and methamphetamine can lead to cardiovascular issues, respiratory problems, neurological damage, and infectious diseases (e.g., HIV, hepatitis).

- Mental Health: Drug use can exacerbate mental health disorders, lead to addiction, and impair cognitive functions and emotional regulation.

- Behavioral Risks: Drug use increases the

risk of risky behaviors, accidents, and violence. It can also lead to legal and social issues.

Prevention and Treatment

- Prevention: Effective prevention strategies include education, early intervention, and community support programs.

- Treatment: Treatment for drug use disorders often involves a combination of behavioral therapies, counseling, and medications tailored to the specific substance used and individual needs.

INTEGRATED APPROACH TO SUBSTANCE USE AND HEALTH

Comprehensive Strategies

Addressing substance use requires a holistic approach that combines prevention, treatment, and support:

Prevention Programs: Community-based programs, school education, and public health campaigns aim to prevent the onset of substance use and educate individuals about its risks.

Treatment and Rehabilitation: Effective treatment involves medical, psychological, and social interventions to support recovery and prevent relapse.

Support Systems: Support from family, friends, and support groups plays a crucial role in recovery and maintaining a substance-free lifestyle.

POLICY AND ENVIRONMENTAL CHANGES

• Regulation: Policies that regulate tobacco

and alcohol sales, promote smoke-free environments, and address prescription drug misuse can contribute to reduced substance use and related health risks.

• Access to Resources: Ensuring access to mental health and addiction services, including counseling and treatment facilities, is essential for supporting individuals affected by substance use disorders.

Conclusion

Substance use, including smoking, alcohol consumption, and drug use, has profound effects on health and longevity. Understanding the risks associated with these behaviors and implementing effective strategies for prevention, treatment, and support are crucial for improving health outcomes and extending life expectancy. The following chapters will further explore the impact of environmental factors, genetic predispositions, and mental health on overall health, providing a comprehensive approach to promoting a longer, healthier life.

ENVIRONMENTAL FACTORS: THE INFLUENCE OF POLLUTION AND HAZARDOUS CONDITIONS

Environmental factors play a crucial role in determining health outcomes and influencing life expectancy. These factors include exposure to pollution, hazardous living conditions, and other environmental hazards. Understanding how these factors impact health is essential for mitigating risks and promoting long-term well-being.

KEY CONCEPTS

➢ Environmental Health: A branch of public health that focuses on how environmental factors affect human health and well-being.

➤ Pollutants: Substances in the environment that can cause harm to human health, including chemicals, particulate matter, and biological agents.

Types of Pollution

1. Air Pollution: Includes pollutants such as particulate matter (PM2.5 and PM10), nitrogen dioxide (NO2), sulfur dioxide (SO2), carbon monoxide (CO), and ozone (O3). Sources include vehicle emissions, industrial processes, and burning of fossil fuels.

2. Water Pollution: Involves contamination of water bodies by harmful substances, including heavy metals, pesticides, and

pathogens. Sources include industrial discharge, agricultural runoff, and inadequate wastewater treatment.

3. Soil Pollution: Caused by the presence of hazardous chemicals in the soil, often due to improper disposal of waste, use of pesticides, and industrial activities.

Health Impacts

1. Respiratory Issues: Air pollution can lead to chronic respiratory conditions such as asthma, chronic bronchitis, and chronic obstructive pulmonary disease (COPD). Long-term exposure increases the risk of lung cancer.

2. Cardiovascular Health: Pollutants like particulate matter and nitrogen dioxide can exacerbate cardiovascular diseases by increasing blood pressure and contributing to the development of atherosclerosis.

3. Neurological Effects: Emerging research suggests that exposure to certain pollutants may affect cognitive function and is associated with neurological disorders such as dementia.

4. Reproductive and Developmental Health: Exposure to pollutants like heavy metals and endocrine disruptors can impact reproductive health, fetal development, and increase the risk of birth defects.

Mitigation and Prevention

- Regulation and Policy: Implementing and enforcing environmental regulations to limit emissions and improve waste management can reduce pollution levels.

- Technological Solutions: Advances in technology, such as cleaner energy sources and pollution control devices, can help reduce environmental pollution.

- Community Actions: Public awareness campaigns, promoting green spaces, and encouraging sustainable practices can contribute to reducing individual and collective exposure to pollutants.

HAZARDOUS LIVING CONDITIONS

Definition and Types

Hazardous living conditions refer to environments that pose significant risks to health and safety. These include:

Inadequate Sanitation: Poor sanitation facilities and lack of clean drinking water can lead to the spread of infectious diseases, such as diarrhea, cholera, and other waterborne illnesses.

Substandard Housing: Poor housing conditions, including inadequate heating, ventilation, and structural integrity, can contribute to health problems such as respiratory infections, lead poisoning, and injuries.

Occupational Hazards: Work environments that expose individuals to harmful substances or unsafe conditions can lead to health issues such as respiratory diseases, cancers, and musculoskeletal disorders.

Health Impacts

1. Infectious Diseases: Inadequate sanitation and poor hygiene can lead to outbreaks of infectious diseases, significantly impacting health and life expectancy.

2. Chronic Health Conditions:Substandard housing can exacerbate chronic conditions, such as asthma and cardiovascular disease, due to mold, poor air quality, and extreme

temperatures.

3. Accidents and Injuries: Unsafe working conditions and poorly maintained living environments increase the risk of accidents and injuries, which can have long-term health implications.

Improving Living Conditions

- Infrastructure Development: Investing in improved sanitation, safe housing, and better infrastructure can significantly enhance living conditions and health outcomes.

- Occupational Safety: Implementing and enforcing workplace safety standards can reduce exposure to hazardous conditions and prevent occupational diseases.

- Community Health Initiatives: Local health initiatives aimed at improving living conditions, such as providing access to clean water and safe housing, play a crucial role in promoting health.

Climate Change and Health

Impact of Climate Change

Climate change affects health through various mechanisms, including:

Extreme Weather Events: Increased frequency and intensity of extreme weather events such as heatwaves, storms, and floods can cause direct health impacts, including heat-related illnesses and injuries.

Vector-Borne Diseases: Changes in climate can alter the distribution of disease vectors, such as mosquitoes and ticks, leading to an increased risk of diseases like malaria, dengue fever, and Lyme disease.

Food Security: Climate change can

impact agricultural production, leading to food shortages and malnutrition.

Adaptation and Resilience

Climate Adaptation: Strategies to adapt to climate change include improving infrastructure to withstand extreme weather, developing early warning systems, and promoting climate-resilient agriculture.

Health Systems Strengthening: Enhancing health systems to better respond to the impacts of climate change, such as improving disease surveillance and healthcare access, is crucial for protecting public health.

POLICY AND PUBLIC HEALTH INTERVENTIONS

Policy Measures

• Environmental Regulations: Governments can implement policies to control pollution, improve environmental standards, and promote sustainable practices.

• Public Health Policies: Integrating environmental health considerations into public health policies can help address the broader determinants of health and improve population health outcomes.

Public Awareness and Education

• Community Engagement: Raising awareness about environmental health issues and promoting community engagement in environmental protection can drive collective action and improve health outcomes.

•Education Programs: Educational programs focusing on environmental health can empower individuals to make informed choices and advocate for healthier environments.

Conclusion:

Environmental factors, including pollution, hazardous living conditions, and climate change, have a profound impact on health and longevity. Addressing these factors through effective regulation, technological innovation, and community engagement is essential for improving health outcomes and promoting a longer, healthier life. The following chapters will further explore how genetic predispositions and mental health contribute to health and longevity, providing a comprehensive approach to understanding and enhancing overall well-being.

CHAPTER SEVEN

GENETIC PREDISPOSITIONS: UNDERSTANDING THE ROLE OF GENETICS IN HEALTH AND LONGEVITY

INTRODUCTION TO GENETIC PREDISPOSITIONS

Genetic predispositions refer to the susceptibility to certain health conditions based on an individual's genetic makeup. Genetics play a crucial role in determining risk factors for various diseases, influencing health outcomes, and contributing to overall longevity. While genetics can predispose individuals to certain conditions, lifestyle and environmental factors also play significant roles.

Genotype: The genetic constitution of an individual, which determines potential health risks and traits.

Phenotype: The observable characteristics or traits of an individual resulting from the interaction between genotype and environment.

HEREDITY AND GENETIC DISORDERS

Inherited Conditions

Genetic disorders are diseases or conditions caused by abnormalities in an individual's DNA. These can be inherited from one or both parents and are categorized into several types:

- Autosomal Dominant Disorders: Conditions caused by a single copy of a mutated gene. Examples include

Huntington's disease and Marfan syndrome.

- Autosomal Recessive Disorders: Conditions requiring two copies of a mutated gene to manifest. Examples include cystic fibrosis and sickle cell anemia.

- X-Linked Disorders: Conditions linked to genes on the X chromosome. Examples include hemophilia and Duchenne muscular dystrophy.

Genetic Testing

Genetic testing can identify mutations associated with inherited conditions and assess risk for certain diseases:

- Diagnostic Testing: Confirms the presence of a genetic disorder in individuals showing symptoms.

- Predictive Testing: Assesses the risk of developing a genetic disorder before symptoms appear.

- Carrier Testing: Determines if an individual carries a gene for an inherited disorder, which can be important for family planning.

THE ROLE OF GENETICS IN COMMON DISEASES

Cardiovascular Diseases

Genetic factors contribute to the risk of cardiovascular diseases such as coronary artery disease, hypertension, and heart failure:

- Familial Hypercholesterolemia: A genetic condition leading to high cholesterol levels and increased risk of heart disease.

- Hypertrophic Cardiomyopathy: A genetic disorder that affects the heart muscle, potentially leading to heart failure.

Cancer

Genetics play a significant role in the risk of

developing certain cancers:

- Hereditary Breast and Ovarian Cancer Syndrome: Caused by mutations in the BRCA1 and BRCA2 genes, increasing the risk of breast and ovarian cancer.

- Lynch Syndrome: A genetic condition increasing the risk of colorectal and other cancers.

Diabetes

Genetic factors contribute to the risk of developing diabetes:

- Type 1 Diabetes: An autoimmune condition with a genetic component that affects insulin production.

- Type 2 Diabetes: A condition influenced by both genetic predisposition and lifestyle factors, including obesity and physical inactivity.

Epigenetics

Epigenetics refers to changes in gene expression that do not involve alterations to the underlying DNA sequence. Environmental factors can influence epigenetic modifications, which can affect health outcomes:

- Lifestyle Factors: Diet, stress, and exposure to toxins can lead to epigenetic changes that influence susceptibility to diseases.

- Developmental Programming: Early life exposures can affect epigenetic markers, potentially leading to long-term health effects.

Personalized Medicine

Personalized medicine uses genetic information to tailor medical treatments and preventive strategies:

- Genetic Profiling: Helps in identifying individual risk factors and choosing appropriate interventions or medications.

- Targeted Therapies: Treatments designed to target specific genetic mutations or abnormalities in diseases such as cancer.

PREVENTIVE MEASURES AND GENETIC COUNSELING

Genetic Counseling

Genetic counseling provides individuals and families with information about genetic conditions and the implications for health:

- Risk Assessment: Evaluates the likelihood of inherited conditions based on family history and genetic testing.

- Decision-Making Support: Helps individuals make informed decisions about testing, treatment options, and family planning.

Lifestyle and Environmental Interventions

Although genetic predispositions can influence health, lifestyle and environmental factors also play a crucial role:

- Healthy Lifestyle Choices: Adopting a balanced diet, regular exercise, and avoiding known risk factors can help mitigate genetic risks.

- Environmental Modifications: Reducing exposure to environmental toxins and maintaining a healthy living environment can help manage genetic predispositions.

FUTURE DIRECTIONS IN GENETIC RESEARCH

Advances in Genomics

• Genome-Wide Association Studies (GWAS): Identifying genetic variants associated with various diseases and traits to improve understanding and treatment.

• Gene Editing Technologies: Innovations like CRISPR-Cas9 offer potential for correcting genetic mutations and treating genetic disorders.

Ethical Considerations

• Privacy and Consent: Ensuring that genetic information is used ethically and with respect to individual privacy and consent.

• Equity and Access: Addressing disparities

in access to genetic testing and personalized medicine to ensure equitable health benefits.

Conclusion

Genetic predispositions play a significant role in determining health risks and influencing longevity. Understanding the interplay between genetics and environmental factors, along with advances in genetic research and personalized medicine, offers opportunities to improve health outcomes and extend life expectancy. The following chapters will explore how mental health, substance use, and environmental factors further impact overall health, providing a comprehensive perspective on achieving a longer and healthier life.

CHAPTER EIGHT

INTEGRATED APPROACHES TO HEALTH: SYNERGIZING FACTORS FOR OPTIMAL LONGEVITY

INTRODUCTION TO INTEGRATED APPROACHES

An integrated approach to health considers the interplay between various factors such as genetics, lifestyle, environment, and mental health. Understanding how these factors interact can lead to more effective strategies for promoting health and extending longevity. This chapter explores how combining insights from different domains can enhance overall well-being and longevity.

Holistic Health: An approach that considers the whole person, including physical, mental, and social aspects, rather than focusing on individual components.

Synergy: The interaction of multiple factors that results in a greater effect than the sum of their individual effects.

Integrating Genetics and Lifestyle Factors

Personalized Health Strategies

Combining genetic information with lifestyle choices can lead to personalized health strategies:

- Genetic Risk Assessment: Identifying genetic predispositions allows for tailored lifestyle modifications and preventive measures. For example, individuals with a genetic predisposition to cardiovascular disease may benefit from targeted dietary and exercise recommendations.

- Lifestyle Interventions: Adopting healthy habits, such as regular exercise, a balanced diet, and stress management, can mitigate genetic risks and improve overall health outcomes.

Case Studies and Examples

- Heart Disease: For individuals with a family history of heart disease, personalized interventions might include specific dietary changes, increased physical activity, and regular cardiovascular screenings.

- Cancer Prevention: Genetic testing for mutations linked to breast cancer can guide preventive measures such as lifestyle modifications and, in some cases, prophylactic surgeries.

Mental Health and Substance Use

Mental health and substance use often interact in complex ways, affecting overall health:

- Dual Diagnosis: Individuals with mental health conditions may be at increased risk for substance use disorders, and vice versa. Integrated treatment approaches that address both mental health and substance use issues are essential for effective management.

- Preventive Measures: Promoting mental well-being through stress management, therapy, and support systems can reduce the risk of substance abuse. Conversely, addressing substance use can improve mental health outcomes.

Comprehensive Treatment Models

- Integrated Care: Coordinating mental health and substance use treatment within a single healthcare framework can improve outcomes. This model includes combined therapy sessions, medication management, and supportive services.

- Community-Based Approaches: Community programs that offer support for both mental health and substance use can enhance access to care and provide holistic support.

ENVIRONMENTAL FACTORS AND HEALTH PROMOTION

Environmental Health Strategies

Addressing environmental factors through integrated health strategies can improve public health:

- Sustainable Practices: Implementing

sustainable practices, such as reducing pollution and promoting green spaces, can enhance environmental quality and support healthier lifestyles.

- Public Health Interventions: Policies and programs aimed at improving living conditions, such as better sanitation and safer housing, contribute to overall health and longevity.

Community and Policy Initiatives

- Collaborative Efforts: Collaborative efforts between government agencies, public health organizations, and community groups can address environmental health challenges effectively.

- Policy Development: Policies that integrate environmental health considerations with public health objectives can promote long-term improvements in health outcomes.

THE ROLE OF TECHNOLOGY AND INNOVATION

❖ Advancements in Healthcare Technology

Technological innovations play a significant role in integrating health factors:

- Telemedicine: Offers access to healthcare services for remote or underserved populations, facilitating integrated care for chronic conditions and mental health issues.

- Wearable Technology: Provides real-time health monitoring, enabling individuals to track lifestyle factors such as physical activity, sleep, and diet.

❖ Future Directions

- Artificial Intelligence: AI can enhance personalized medicine by analyzing large datasets to identify health trends and tailor interventions.

- Genomic Medicine: Advances in genomics may lead to more precise and individualized approaches to health, integrating genetic information with lifestyle and environmental factors.

Implementing Integrated Health Strategies

❖ Personal Health Plans

Developing a personalized health plan involves integrating various factors:

• Assessment: Evaluate genetic risks, lifestyle habits, and environmental exposures.

• Customization: Create a tailored plan that includes dietary recommendations, exercise routines, mental health support, and preventive measures.

• Monitoring: Regularly review and adjust the plan based on changes in health status and emerging research.

❖ Healthcare System Approaches

• Coordinated Care Models: Healthcare systems should implement models that integrate multiple aspects of health, including preventive care, chronic disease management, and mental health services.

• Patient-Centered Care: Focusing on the individual needs and preferences of patients can improve engagement and outcomes.

Conclusion

An integrated approach to health recognizes the complex interplay between genetics, lifestyle, environment, and mental health. By synergizing these factors, individuals and healthcare systems can develop more effective strategies for promoting health and extending longevity.

This comprehensive approach not only enhances individual well-being but also fosters a healthier society. The insights from this chapter emphasize the importance of holistic health strategies in achieving optimal health outcomes and providing a foundation for future advancements in health and longevity.

REFERENCES

Global Burden of Disease Study 2019 Collaborators (2020). The Lancet.

Comprehensive data on global

chronic disease burden, including

cardiovascular diseases, diabetes,

and cancer.

American Heart Association (2021). Circulation. Updated statistics on

cardiovascular disease and stroke

prevalence, risk factors, and

outcomes.

International Diabetes Federation (2021).

IDF Diabetes Atlas. Detailed

global and regional data on diabetes prevalence and management strategies.

U.S. Department of Health and Human Services (2020). Centers for Disease Control and Prevention. A comprehensive review of the health effects of smoking and tobacco use.

GBD Alcohol Collaborators (2018). The Lancet. Analysis of alcohol use's impact on global health and disease burden.

Koob, G.F., & Volkow, N.D. (2016). Neuropsychopharmacology. Discusses neurobiological

mechanisms of drug addiction
and treatment strategies.

Brook, R.D., Rajagopalan, S., Pope, C.A., et
al. (2010). Circulation. Reviews the impact
of air pollution on
cardiovascular health.

World Health Organization (2021). WHO
Report. Outlines health impacts of
climate change and adaptation
strategies.

Kumar, A., & Kaur, M. (2018).
Environmental Science and Pollution
Research.

Reddy, S., Koyanagi, S., Bhattacharya, S., et
al. (2015). Cardiovascular Research.
Reviews genetic and epigenetic
factors contributing to

cardiovascular diseases.

Miki, Y., Swensen, J., Shattuck-Eidens, D., et al. (1994). Science. Identifies BRCA1 and BRCA2 genes and their association with breast and ovarian cancer.

Visscher, P.M., Brown, M.A., McCarthy, M.I., Yang, J. (2012). Nature.

Murray, C.J.L., Vos, T., Lozano, R., et al. (2013). The Lancet Psychiatry. Overview of mental health disorders, substance use, and their interaction.

Hoge, M.A., Morris, J.A., Hohman, M., et al. (2014).American Journal of Psychiatry.

Katz, D.L., & Meller, S. (2014). American Journal of Lifestyle Medicine.

Highlights the impact of lifestyle

and behavioral changes on disease

prevention and longevity.